EASY AGING:

20 SCIENTIFIC, PROVEN HABITS

BY

MAGGIE HANKAMP

Table of Contents

INTRODUCTION:

At age 71, I feel I am able to give some great advice because I have been a life-long learner and reader of so many texts. I also attend many self help conferences because I like learning.

I face both an active future and the realization that death waits nearby. I do not fear death because my days and nights have been filled with love, adventure, learning, joy, and success as well as failures that taught me how to progress. So these habits are habits I use frequently, some every day.

May you read these 20 HABITS, pick out several to practice, be fortified, feel that all is well, and realize at any age we can improve our lives, change our brains with neuroplasticity, and make our lives easier and more fun!

EMAIL me at HANKAMP@GMAIL.COM if you feel strongly about any entry. Even if you just want to talk or want encouragement, email me.

Of course, if you say I have missed some habits, sure, please tell me and I will write another book for that addition.

I also feel we are learning so much about health and longevity and excellent aging practices,, each year there will be new additions to these habits.

Love, Hugs, Laughter to every cell of your body!,

Maggie Hankamp

Spring Hill, FL

February, 2019

Revised November 2019

CHAPTER ONE
HABIT: BREATHE

OK, OK, We are breathing now or you would not be reading this. Although, I often feel the presence of many members of my family looking over my shoulder, that is not the case here.

So, our breath is the most important aspect of our lives. We breathe to give oxygen and sustenance to each and every cell in our body. We breathe to help all of our bodily functions take place. We breathe to feel good. We breathe to let our fears and grief go. We breathe when we laugh hardily. We breathe to live and enjoy this life.

So, HOW are you breathing right now? Take time to feel your breath. Take time to measure how long your in breath and out breath is. Right now, make a note of that measurement.

Pay attention to your breath. Is your breath short and panting like a puppy dog, or is it long and slow and smooth like a slowly flowing river?

Stop what you are doing several times a day. Pay attention to your breath. Once you realize how your breath is moving, then do one of the following:

If breath is slow and smoothly going along, then continue with that habit. Enjoy the sense of calm and relaxation that this breath gives you.

If your breath is short and panting like a puppy, then take time and stop what you are doing. Make the effort to breathe in as long as is comfortable. Then take the time to breathe out with the same amount of time. Do this just for a minute. Then go about your business.

This habit works best if you can create several "automatic nudges." Whenever the phone rings, try to practice breathing. Or, practice breathing before each meal and notice how your meal tastes afterwards.

BONUS CHAPTER ONE HABIT: BREATHE:

ONCE YOU BECOME AWARE OF HOW YOU ARE BREATHING, MAKE IT A HABIT ALSO TO BREATHE LONGER ON THE EXHALE THAN ON THE INHALE.

FOR EXAMPLE, IF YOU COUNT THAT YOU BREATHE IN TO THE COUNT OF FOUR, AIM TO MAKE YOUR EXHALE TO THE COUNT OF EIGHT OR LONGER.

THIS HABIT ACTIVATES YOUR PARASYMPATHETIC NERVOUS SYSTEM. YOU REDUCE YOUR STRESS WITH THESE LONGER EXHALES AND YOU CHANGE SEVERAL OTHER IMPORTANT HEALTH FACTORS, TOO..

CHAPTER TWO
HABIT: STRETCH:

What fun! Here is a habit easily achieved from the warmth and comfort of your bed. Have you ever taken time to really stretch before getting out of bed?

Or, late in the evening or whenever you are ready for a long sleep, have you taken the time to really stretch your body and enjoy that feeling?

So, how does one do a stretch?

You could begin in the morning by raising your arms up as high as they go overhead. And from there feel the pull as you reach as high as you are able. While reaching high, do an action of pulling your legs downward and even, if not painful, point your toes. So, act like a spring, see yourself lengthening out as you do this action for a few seconds.

At night, before sleeping, focus again on your arms and hands and feet. Aim again to have your feet and arms pulled apart like a spring. Hold this position for several seconds. Once you have gotten in the habit of stretching, then hold the stretch for a longer time.

Again, create a reminder that says, "Now, I stretch for two seconds before getting out of bed." And, at nighttime, say again and add this to your nighttime routine: "I will stretch to my fullest and feel that sense of relaxation overcome me."

BONUS CHAPTER TWO HABIT: STRETCH:

DURING THE DAY, SEE IF YOU MIGHT LIKE THAT SAME SENSE OF WELL BEING THAT THE MORNING AND EVENING STRETCH GIVE YOU.

WHILE STANDING AT THE SINK WASHING DISHES OR PREPARING FOOD, HOLD ONTO THE COUNTER, PULL THE NECK AND FEET PART. FEEL THE SPINE LENGTHEN AND RELAX.

OR, WHILE SITTING WATCHING TV, LIFT YOUR ARMS AND STRETCH YOUR FEEET OUT IN FRONT OF YOU. FEEL THE EFFECT THAT THIS GIVES TO YOUR SPINE AND TO YOUR BREATHING AND TO YOUR FLEXIBILITY.

CHAPTER THREE
HABIT: POSTURE:

Now, I have practiced yoga since I was 27 years old. I began by taking an adult education course through the Arlington Central School District adult programs. I joined the class with my sister, Terri. I enjoyed the effects on my spine and shoulders. I felt so good. I thought I knew good posture. Yet at age 71 I now have improved remarkably on my posture.

A BIG thank you to Barb at the Suncoast YMCA for her lessons on how to actually keep a good posture.

Barb explains how to keep your sternum reaching up toward the cove. Your sternum is your breastbone in the center of your chest. The cove is that area where the wall touches the ceiling.

Try this habit now:

If you are standing on the NYC subway, hold onto the pole, allow your sternum to rise to the point where the wall of the subway car meets the top of the subway car.. Let your shoulder blades move inwards on your back.Relax there and breathe.

If you are sitting while reading this, put your hand on your sternum, feel it reach up to the cove. Feel your shoulder blades reach inwards towards your spine. Relax and breathe there.

No need to lift shoulders, no need to do any other actions, just feel this posture habit allowing your shoulder blades to drop and rest.

BONUS CHAPTER THREE HABIT: POSTURE:

ONCE YOU FEEL THIS STERNUM TO COVE GOOD POSTURE,YOU WOULD LIKE TO FEEL THIS ALL THE TIME. THIS GREAT HABIT SHOWS UP IN BETTER DIGESTION, EASIER WALKING, AND IN A POWERFUL AND CALMER SENSE OF SELF-ESTEEM.

HOW MAY WE ADD THIS HABIT TO OUR DAY-LONG BEHAVIOR?

BECOME AWARE OF HOW YOU ARE STANDING OR SITTING. START WITH ONE ACTION YOU DO OFTEN:I SUGGEST THAT A GOOD PLACE TO START USING THIS POSTURE HABIT IS WITH OUR CELL PHONE USAGE.

CAN YOU STILL SEE THE SCREEN IF YOU PRACTICE THIS POS-TURE HABIT?

 CAN YOU BREATHE EASIER WITH THIS HABIT?

CHAPTER FOUR HABIT: TAPPING/EMOTIONAL FREEDOM TECHNIQUE:

I am grateful that I learned this habit over 10 years ago. Tapping has changed my life in so many ways. You ask, "What is Tapping/Emotional Freedom Technique?"

Tapping is a method of lessening stress and making changes in our brain pathways so we do not respond to people or events or dramas in the same old fashion. In Tapping, we gently yet firmly tap or press or hold various acupressure points on our body, using Traditional Chinese Medicine points (TCM). We can use this habit to reduce pain, eliminate fears and phobias, change our outlook to more joy, and grow in health, spirituality, and freedom.

So, let's tap on the fear of getting older:

Begin by tapping repeatedly with two or three fingers of one hand on the fleshy outside edge (the karate point) of the other hand and saying: "Even though I am so fearful of getting older, I deeply and completely love and accept myself and my fears." Tap the karate point 3 times saying this.

Then, tap on the following points (ONE ROUND) while using a reminder phrase such as "Getting older"

- Top of Head
- Beginning of Eyebrow

- Side of Eye
- Under Eye
- Under Nose
- Under Lips
- Collarbone Point
- Under arms
- Bottom of Rib Cage
- Tap Wrists Together

Continue tapping until you feel a lessening of your fear of getting older.

Even better, tap and speak about a particular pain or fear, just one single one at a time, you might have, such as "Even though I fear the loss of mobility that I may experience, I deeply and completely love and accept myself."

BONUS CHAPTER FOUR HABIT: TAPPING/EFT:

TAPPING FOR NO REASON.

YES, YOU HAVE THAT RIGHT: TAPPING FOR NO REASON IS A GREAT WAY TO ESTABLISH THE GOOD EFFECTS OF STRESS REDUCTION EVEN IF NO WORDS NOR ANY EVENTS COME TO MIND.

SO, EACH MORNING AND EACH EVENING, DO ONE

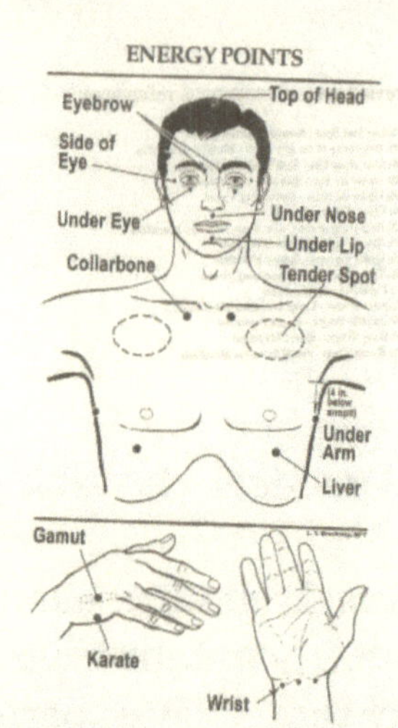

ROUND OF TAPPING AND FEEL THE STRESS LESSEN.

CHAPTER FIVE HABIT: MORNING HABIT:

So, stop and think, what habits would make your day go better?

We have talked about breathing and stretching and posture and tapping, all of which improve our feeling of well-being. For sure, start your day with these habits. And then add one other habit to our mornings: Intending how our day will go.

Each morning our best shot at having a happy, healthy, joy-filled day is by setting an intention for that to happen.

Intention setting may be done by simply saying:

"Today I intend to have the healthiest and happiest day ever." Or, take one of your pressing jobs and say, "Today I intend to do the best ever work at ________________."

Regardless of how you set your intention, make it a daily habit to use the early hours of any day to predict and plan how your day will unfold.

BONUS CHAPTER FIVE: MORNING HABIT:

EARLY IN THE MORNING, GET A PEN AND WRITE DOWN FIVE FEARS AND/OR WORRIES ABOUT THE UPCOMING DAY.

USE THIS LIST TO MAKE UP THE BEST INTENTION FOR THIS DAY EVER.

"TODAY I PLAN TO DO MY BEST TO WORK ON _______________."

"TODAY I KNOW I CAN BE SUCCESSFUL AT _____________________."

"TODAY THE FEAR OF _______________ WILL HELP ME MOVE AHEAD TO DO MORE AMAZING THINGS."

"REGARDLESS OF MY WORRIES ABOUT THIS DAY, I PLAN TO FEEL GOOD AND JOYFUL AND RELEASE ANY WORRIES THAT DO NOT HELP ME GROW TO BE A BETTTER PERSON.

CHAPTER SIX HABIT: EVENING HABIT:

Have you been reading and hearing all that information about SLEEP being the way to health and renewal? Did you realize your stomach cells, for example, rebuild and renew overnight as we rest?

This evening habit is one that can be used so easily. This habit takes only a few minutes. It is so easy you may think, "No way is that going to help me get a good night's sleep!"

But I have been using this successfully and find my sleep is great and uninterrupted, except for bathroom visits.... :-)

So, here it goes:

As bedtime comes on, take a pen and a piece of paper, not a computer nor cell phone since their light may interrupt your best sleep:.

Write down everything that is on your mind:
work that needs to be done
events that are upcoming
things you wanted to finish today
family complaints
money worries
job concerns
health concerns, etc.

Once all is written down, take a moment to breathe in and out.

Then say to yourself, " All of these can be takencare of at another time. I am letting these go; I am allowing myself to have the best night's sleep ever."

Then either rip that paper up and throw it away in the trash or fold this paper up and put it away.

Go get that good night's sleep!

BONUS CHAPTER SIX HABIT: EVENING HABIT:

WHEN HAVE YOU LAST TAKEN A SLOW AND ENJOYABLE BATH? ADD SOME ESSENTIAL OIL, LAVENDER, FOR EXAMPLE, OR EPSOM SALT FOR CLEARING YOUR AURA AND HELPING YOU RELIEVE MUSCLE PAINS.

A BATH IS A TIME OF RELAXATION, PEACE, CALM AND EVEN, AS OFTEN AS I TAKE A BATH, A CHANCE TO RECHARGE AND KNOW WHAT YOU WANT IN LIFE.

TRY THIS HABIT WHENEVER OVERWHELMED BY LIFE, I GUARANTEE IT WILL HELP YOU GET THE BEST SLEEP!

CHAPTER SEVEN
HABIT: MASSAGE:

I hear my friends and neighbors laughing and saying, "Of course Maggie will recommend massage because she is a licensed massage therapist!"

BUT, have you read the research about massage lessening so many problems and so many stresses? And, please think, the cost for a massage may help you avoid medical expenses for stress-related dis-eases.

So, here goes: You deserve the best massage therapist for your needs.

Ask friends or family if they know a reliable massage therapist. Check professional associations/people such as:

- AMBP: Associated Bodywork & Massage Professionals
- AMTA: American Massage Therapy Association
- Your own state licensing department which lists those professionals who are licensed and trained and continuing their professional education
- your family doctor

If you have never enjoyed a massage before, take the time to visit a therapist and discuss your needs. See what the setting is like, feel if you are comfortable with the therapist, and ask any questions you may have.

BONUS CHAPTER SEVEN HABIT: MASSAGE:

AHH, I AM LAUGHING, I WONDERED IF YOU WOULD THINK THERE COULD NOT BE A BONUS FOR MASSAGE.

WELL, THERE IS:

GO TO YOUTUBE.COM. WRITE IN THE SEARCH BOX "JAPANESE FACIAL MASSAGE."

FOLLOW ALONG AND LEARN HOW TO GENTLY AND FIRMLY MASSAGE YOUR OWN FACE WHILE ALSO OFTEN DECREASING WRINKLE LINES.

ENJOY THIS VERY CALMING AND RESTFUL SELF CARE ROUTINE!

CHAPTER EIGHT
HABIT: REFLEXOLOGY:

The cat is out of the bag; I told you in the last chapter about facial massage.

Learn about total body massage using reflexology.

Based on Traditional Chinese Medicine, reflexology is the massaging of the hands or the feet or the ears or the tongue to help the entire body relax and allow the body's focus on healing to come out.

Let's begin with hand reflexology. You may get the chart for hand reflexology on a google search.

Start by massaging gently yet firmly all around and up and down each finger, including your thumb.

Then, using your thumb on opposite hand or even two fingers of the opposite hand, gently begin massaging the entire palm, going in a horizontal direction first and including the side of the palm. If any spot is sore, stop and gently massage that even longer.

Then, change directions. Use the thumb or two fingers to move up and down vertically. Again, if any spot is sore, stop a moment and gently massage longer.

I have found this reflexology of the hands works great. I used it recently on an overseas flight of nine hours to keep any swelling down in my ankles or feet. It worked wonders, all was well!

BONUS CHAPTER EIGHT HABIT: REFLEXOLOGY:

THIS BONUS FOLLOWS WHAT YOU HAVE JUST WORKED ON WITH A FOCUS ON YOUR EARS.

YOU MAY WORK ON BOTH EARS AT ONCE IF YOU ARE NOT DRIVING NOR OPERATING HEAVY EQUIPMENT. :-)

GENTLY AND FIRMLY BEGIN HOLDING THE TOP OF THE EARS IN BETWEEN YOUR THUMB AND INDEX POINTER FINGER. MOVE THE THUMB AND FINGER OUTWARD PRESSING ON THE EAR AND UNFURLING THE EDGE OF THE EAR.

THEN, MOVE VERY, VERY SLOWLY DOWN THE EAR. CONTINU-ING THE SAME ACTION OF GENTLY PULLING AND MOVING THE THUMB AND FINGER OUTWARD ON THE EAR.

AFTER REACHING THE BOTTOM OF THE EAR, THE END POINT, GO AND BEGIN AGAIN AT THE TOP OF THE EAR.

FEEL THE CALM!

IF YOU ARE FEELING VERY ADVENTURESOME, CONTINUE WITH ONE FINGER THAT GENTLY PRESSES INTO THE FLESHY, CURVING AREAS OF THE OUTSIDE OF THE EAR.

CHAPTER NINE HABIT: TIME WITH FRIENDS

This is a very interesting habit.

I wonder if people do realize that time, real quality time spent with friends, can be a health advantage?

The British National Health Service has declared loneliness as one of the pressing health factors across all of Britain.

I have a feeling it is also an essential component to health here in the United States. If you are missing friendships, it is bad for your own health.

So, you say, "All my friends have died." that sure is unfortunate......I am sorry for your suffering.

However, what is wrong with making a friend who is 18 years old or 35 years old or 63 years old?

Also, consider the statement, IN ORDER TO GAIN A FRIEND, YOU MUST BE A FRIEND FIRST. What have you done today that may make a new friend or renew an old friendship?

- Have you reconnected with an old friend by calling and listening to them and hearing is going on in their life? Or
- Have you smiled at another person at the post office or at the grocery store who is waiting in line for service? Or
- Have you joined meetup.com to connect with people

who enjoy the same activities and outlets as you do? Or
- Have you visited a church or temple or synagogue that would have similar people with similar values? Or
- Have you volunteered at some activity or some place that you value and/or enjoy greatly?

The choices are endless. It is our choice to be alone or to be with other people.

BONUS CHAPTER NINE HABIT: TIME WITH FRIENDS:

ALL OF MODERN TECHNOLOGY, CELL PHONES, COMPUTER, TV, ALEXA, HAVE NOT EASED OUR LONELINESS.

TODAY, GO TO LUNCH WITH SOMEONE AND TURN YOUR CELL PHONE OFF, OFF, OFF, UNLESS YOUR WIFE IS EXPECTING A BABY AND IS DUE ANY MINUTE.

OR, TODAY, GO SHOPPING AND TALK WITH THE SALESPERSON WITH CELL PHONE OFF, OFF, OFF.

OR, IF TALKING WITH SOMEONE ON THE CELL PHONE, LISTEN ONLY, NO MULTITASKING NEEDED.

CHAPTER TEN HABIT: TIME WITH FAMILY:

Here family can mean your family of birth or also your family of choice. Family here is related to Habit Eight, but includes a stronger personal and loving and compassionate element. Family is "ohana," those people who love you no matter what and love you totally unconditionally

Some of our families may be difficult and challenging to be with on a regular basis. I read where in Japan it has become culturally acceptable and/or fashionable to "Rent a Family" for an event or for special occasions. So, for a Cherry Blossom Picnic, rent a Grandmother and Grandfather and/or maybe even a grandchild or two. Complete your own idea of family in that way; however, the worry is what happens when that commercial relationship ends.

So, who is your family? With whom do you look forward to talking and spending time with and enjoying holidays? Do not decide right now. Think and feel your way into this answer.

THEN, only then, see what arrangements can be made to enjoy time with those people you label as family. Understand what limits this family grouping may have. Be aware that you may want to make accommodations that will honor your own needs first.

So, if a family member is difficult to deal with, remember CHAPTER ONE HABIT, and use your breath to keep yourself calm and focused on compassion. I myself find that the CHAPTER FOUR

HABIT OF TAPPING/EFT has eased many a stressful situation when family members do or say or act in ways that are hurtful or insensitive or uncaring. The neuroplasticity of the brain encourages me to have a new way of looking at this person or event.

Remember that we CHOSE our parents for a purpose. We are meant to learn something from this relationship. We are meant to grow through this relationship.

Remember that Ancient Romans paid to have someone follow them around all day, just to agitate them and make them grow emotionally and spiritually.

BONUS CHAPTER TEN HABIT: TIME WITH FAMILY:

HMMM, MIGHT HAVE BEEN HINTED AT IN CHAPTER EIGHT HABIT........HAVE YOU EVER TURNED YOUR CELL PHONE OFF AS YOU ENTERED YOUR HOME?

YOUR HOME IS YOUR SPACE OF REST AND RENEWAL AND LOVE.

YOUR HOME HAS THE MOST IMPORTANT PEOPLE IN THE WORLD TO YOU.

PLEASE SHOW THEM THAT RESPECT AND HONOR THEM AS THE MOST IMPORTANT PEOPLE IN YOUR LIFE:
- **LISTEN TO WHAT THEY ARE SAYING.**
- **MAYBE PLAY A GAME.**
- **MAYBE GO OUT FOR A WALK AFTER DINNER.**
- **MAYBE SING A SONG.**
- **MAYBE PLAY AN INSTRUMENT.**

CHAPTER ELEVEN
HABIT: BODY SCAN:

Have you ever scanned your own body? No machinery needed. Just an attention on each part of your body and an acceptance of what is going on in your body.

Why should we do this?

Well, each time you visit a doctor, you get maybe 5 to 10 minutes worth of time. You often see the Physician's Assistant more than you see the doctor. I personally have never met the assigned doctor; I see the Physician's Assistant, the PA seems sensible to me. :-)

YOU are the architect of your own body. You can spend three hours if you like, scanning and feeling what is going on in your own body.

To begin, I like starting at my toes. Feel free to start at your head if that appeals to you.

Say to yourself and sense how each part of the body feels: "How are you doing, toes?" Continue on, with the entire foot; "How are you doing, feet?" Then, to ankle, "How are you doing, ankles?" Then to calves and shins: "How are you doing, calves and shins?"

If you find a pain or discomfort any place, make note of that. Come back and place your hand, if possible on that area. Say to that place of discomfort or pain, "I love you. What do you want to tell me?" Be open and listen to any answers.

BONUS CHAPTER ELEVEN HABIT: BODY SCAN:

YOU WILL BENEFT FROM REVIEWING CHAPTER 4 HABIT ON TAPPING. THEN, AS YOU SCAN YOUR BODY, MAKE NOTE AS ABOVE OF ANY DISCOMFORT OR PAIN.

NOTE ALSO HOW HIGH ON THE PAIN SCALE THIS FEELING IS, 0 IS FOR NO PAIN, 5 IS MODERATE PAIN, 10 IS OW, OW, OW, BEST CALL DOCTOR. AND CALL, AS NEEDED, WHILE TAPPING.

THEN TAP ALONG ON ONE ITEM OF PAIN ONLY.

START WITH THE KARATE POINT. "EVEN THOUGH I HAVE THIS PAIN AT LEVEL _____, I DEEPLY AND COMPLETELY LOVE AND ACCEPT AND FORGIVE MYSELF AND MY PAIN."

TAP THROUGH THE POINTS: TOP OF HEAD, EYEBROW, SIDE OF EYE, UNDER EYE, UNDER NOSE, UNDER LIPS, COLLAR BONE, UNDERARMS, BOTTOM OF RIB CAGE, AND WRISTS TOGETHER. BREATHE AND DRINK SOME WATER AS NEEDED.

CONTINUE TAPPING UNTIL YOUR PAIN OR

DISCOMFORT IS TO A "0" OR "1" LEVEL.

CHAPTER TWELVE HABIT: YEARLY PHYSICAL:

I hear you, not everyone is blessed with this option. If you have the comfort and back up of a medical plan that allows you to get a once yearly physical, fabulous! If not insured, please ask and see if there are any public health clinics in your area.

Go for it! Write down any concerns ahead of time so your short time with the Nurse or the Physician's Assistant or, perhaps with a doctor, might be used to best advantage. Listen and learn. Be attentive to what is suggested.

Ask yourself, "Does this suggestion seem reasonable?" For any suggested tests or suggested treatments, ask where and how to find out more about the options.

If tests and/or treatments seem reasonable, then find out the costs and/or ask, "Are these covered by my medical coverage that I have?"

Do not be a pushover for medications!

Many doctors have a reputation as "Pill Pushers" for good reason. IF YOU ARE TAKING OVER THREE PRESCRIPTION MEDICATIONS, PLEASE ASK YOUR PHARMACIST FOR A PROFESSIONAL REVIEW OF THE INTERACTIONS. Sadly, overmedication is totally OUR FAULT as consumers of medical care.

WE go to the doctor looking for IMMMEDIATE cure. Instead realize that any condition took a while to come on; it most likely needs some time to clear itself up.

BONUS CHAPTER TWELVE HABIT: YEARLY PHYSICAL:

RESEARCH SHOWS THAT FOOD IS THE FIRST MEDICINE. THAT'S RIGHT, FOOD IS THE FIRST MEDICINE. DID YOU HEAR ME, FOOD IS THE FIRST MEDICINE!

SO, WRITE DOWN WHAT YOU EAT AND WHEN. KEEP A FOOD JOURNAL. SO IF NURSE ASKS YOU DO YOU EAT FRUITS AND VEGETABLES, YOU MAY ANSWER TRUTHFULLY, "ONLY WHEN I EAT CHINESE FOOD", OR " YES, I HAVE FIVE SERVINGS EACH DAY."

OF COURSE, IT GOES WITHOUT SAYING:

- **STOP SMOKING! TAPPING HELPS WITH THAT...........**
- **STOP EATING ALL SUGAR AND WHITE BREADS........**
- **STOP OR REDUCE ALCOHOL CONSUMPTION! TAPPING HELPS........**
- **MOVE YOUR BODY MORE!**
- **LEARN STRESS REDUCTION TECHNIQUES SUCH AS TAPPING**
- **A SECRET, ALL 20 HABITS PRESENTED HERE, AND MOST ESPECIALLY CHAPTER FOUR HABIT: TAPPING, WILL HELP YOU LESSEN STRESS.**

CHAPTER THIRTEEN
HABIT: DENTAL
CHECK UPS:

The health of our teeth appears to be directly related to our heart health......bad teeth are often inflamed and can be harming our whole body. And bad gums, yes, they also need care and respect so the rest of the body is as healthy as the gums are.

Now, I grew up with a father and mother who believed, "What a miracle dentures are! There is no need to worry about teeth. We can get a new set of dentures and all is well." So, in our family, teeth were allowed to be pulled out at the drop of a hat.

Well that idea has now been proven false...... No matter how or what needs to be done, it is best to keep as many of your own teeth as possible. Do not be fooled by denture ads on the tv or in the newspaper from the quick dental shops, "Overnight success to a great smile."

Not true!

Find a dentist who helps you overcome any fears you might have remaining from your childhood or from prior dental work. Here, remember CHAPTER FOUR HABIT TAPPING helps lessen those old fears and associations. Find a dental clinic where the dentists will work with you and save as many teeth as possible.

And, if you have children, I recommend right before their teenage years, have the dentist coat their teeth so cavities will be less likely to form. An expense, but in my opinion well worth the time because it adds much life to your children's teeth.

BONUS CHAPTER THIRTEEN HABIT: DENTAL CHECK UPS:

THIS BONUS SEEMS TOO EASY: BRUSH FOR TWO MINUTES. MAKE SURE YOU AND YOUR CHILDREN BRUSH YOUR/THEIR TEETH AT LEAST TWICE DAILY FOR TWO FULL MINUTES EACH TIME.

MANY DENTISTS ARE NOW HANDING OUT TWO-MINUTE TIMERS TO EACH CLIENT BECAUSE THIS SIMPLE HABIT HELPS TEETH STAY THEIR CLEANEST AND WHITEST FOR THE LONGEST TIME. SO, THE NEED FOR DENTAL REPAIRS GOES DOWN BECAUSE YOU SPEND THE TIME AND EFFORT TO CLEAN YOUR OWN TEETH.

HERE, I SUGGEST MY OWN PERSONAL BIAS AS A BONUS HABIT: BUY A SIMPLE WATER FLOSSER.

USE A WATER FLOSSER ONCE OR TWICE DAILY. YOU WILL BE PLEASED AT THE SENSE OF CLEANLINESS YOU WILL FEEL IN YOUR MOUTH AND GUMS.

OF COURSE, NOTHING IS WRONG WITH THE DAILY USE OF FLOSS. SOMETIMES FLOSS BECOMES MORE DIFFICULT TO USE AS YOU AGE AND HAVE A MORE CHALLENGING TIME AT HOLDING THIN FLOSS.

CHAPTER FOURTEEN
HABIT: LAUGH:

Children are so free with laughter and fun. We adults laugh so little. We do not want to laugh at the struggles or problems of other people. We want to learn how to laugh for no reason and to regain the free and light-hearted sense children are blessed with enjoying.

Laughter Yoga is an easy way to learn laughter for no reason. Laughter Yoga gives us a way to become more relaxed and flexible and enjoy life more. Laughter Yoga is a stress reduction technique, so in addition to laughing you may find yourself crying as you release a long held grief or stress. Dr. Madan Kataria is the originator and creator of Laughter Yoga International.

I was blessed to be trained by one of Dr. Kataria's very best teachers, Dr. Caroline Meeks, known professionally as "Dr. Funshine." Thank you, Dr. Funshine, for all of your Laughter Yoga classes at Mission Bay Park, San Diego, CA, and your Laughter Yoga work that helped so many people of all ages!

Laughter Yoga may be practiced at home. But, LAUGHTER YOGA IS SO MUCH MORE FUN AND FREEING TO PRACTICE IN A GROUP! I Suggest you ask your local YMCA or exercise facility if they teach laughter yoga or would be willing to hold classes.

I want you to have an idea how this works: here is an idea for at home practice, have you ever worked at a big belly laugh for no reason? Find a quiet space in your home or sit in your car or gather with a like-minded friend or two. Start with just a little hee hee laughter noise and shaking of your belly. Allow the noise to get louder; allow the shaking of your belly to become more lively.

At first practice belly laughter for only a half a minute. Feel how it affects your mood and sense of lightness.

Then, add a longer practice time to your belly laughter. All wonders, you feel great after such a practice. So imagine what a group exercise like this would feel like, Bliss!

BONUS CHAPTER FOURTEEN HABIT: LAUGHTER:

MY DEAR FRIEND MIKE IS A VETERAN WHO GETS <u>THE AMERICAN LEGION</u> MAGAZINE. ON THE LAST PAGE IS A GOOD GROUP OF JOKES. HE READS THESE OUTLOUD AND WE HAVE SUCH FUN LAUGHING OUT LOUD AND ENJOYING A NEEDED BREAK FROM SERIOUSNESS.

ALSO, THINK ABOUT SUBSCRIBING TO WWW.A-JOKEADAY.COM. WHY NOT START YOUR DAY WITH SOME CLEAN HUMOR?

AS A LONG TERM EDUCATOR, I WOULD TEACH MY STUDENTS A JOKE. I ASKED THEM TO TELL THE JOKE AT THE DINNER TABLE THAT NIGHT. FOR ALL OF US, THE RECALL POWER TO TELL A JOKE IS A GREAT MEMORY JOB FOR OUR BRAINS. TRY REMEMBERING A JOKE THAT MAKES YOU LAUGH.

CHAPTER FIFTEEN
HABIT: READ:

Reading is a fun method of relaxation. Reading is also a way to learn more painlessly. Reading takes you away from the problems and worries of your everyday life. Reading gives you new worlds to appreciate.

Even five minutes a day of reading some worthwhile material will give you unbelievable rewards. The following titles are some of my favorites over the years:

- John E. Sarnow. <u>Healing Back Pain Naturally, The Mind-Body Connection</u>: Reading this book saved my life and my back thirty plus years ago. Sarnow helped me remove any need for surgery and prescription drugs by teaching my how my mind and my body connected.
- Don Miguel Ruiz. <u>The Four Agreements:</u> I often re-read Don Miguel's simple yet life changing advice: Be impeccable with your word; Do not take anything personally; Always do your best; Do not make assumptions. Life becomes easy!
- Gary Craig. <u>The EFT Manual</u>: Thank you, Gary, for this work about tapping acupressure points which leads to emotional freedom. I use tapping daily. I understand more and more how neuroplasticity enables me to grow mentally and spiritually. Tapping has allowed me to embrace life.

BONUS HAPTER FIFTEEN HABIT: READ:

SOME OF THE FUN TRIPS I MADE WITH MY CHILDREN HAD A BOOK ON TAPE PLAYING. WE ENJOYED FICTION STORIES OR FAMOUS COMEDIANS' ACTS. WE OFTEN FELT UNABLE TO GET OUT OF THE CAR IF A GOOD PART IN THE STORY HAD COME UP, YET WE HAD REACHED OUR DESTINATION. MEMORIES OF LISTENING TO HENNY YOUNGMAN'S OR JACK BENNY'S DRY HUMOR STILL MAKE ME LAUGH TODAY.

SO, HOW CAN YOU ENJOY STORIES: BY PLAYING THEM ON A CD PLAYER OR LISTENING TO THEM IN YOUR CAR.

YOUR LOCAL LIBRARY HAS A WIDE ASSORTMENT OF FICTION AND NONFICTION STORIES. GET YOUR FREE LIBRARY CARD TODAY AND START CHECKING THESE RESOURECES OUT NOW.

OR, ALEXA READS US STORIES, OR, AUDIBLE.COM ALSO EN-COURAGES READING BY AUDIO.......SO NO EXCUSES ABOUT FINISHING THAT BOOK. LISTEN TO THAT BOOK WHILE YOU COMMUTE. OR, LISTEN ON YOUR LUNCH HOUR FROM YOUR CELL PHONE. OR, HAVE YOUR WHOLE FAMILY JOIN IN BY A READING OR LISTENING TIME EACH NIGHT. A FABULOUS HABIT FOR ALL!

CHAPTER SIXTEEN
HABIT: MOVE:

I learned yoga asanas, postures, at age 27. I have been lucky to have used a morning practice through these intervening 45 plus years.

In addition, before joining the Peace Corps to volunteer in Ukraine, 2010-2012, I became a yoga student at Mount Madonna, Watsonville, California. The teachers there had us work on asana, breathing, and best posture using a vinyasa yoga, a more strenuous form of yoga. I graduated with a strong teaching ethic.

I took those yoga lessons over to Ukraine and taught yoga at my site. It was a good way for me to learn the melodic Ukrainian language; it was a fun way to introduce myself to the town and to the college students there in town.

And, now, yoga practice is my early morning go to. Even if I only do the sunrise practice, I have gotten those muscles moving. Is yoga the only exercise to do?

ANY MOVEMENT helps! Get a pedometer and be serious about making those 10,000 steps each day. Or, when you are still in bed, begin a series of movements to flex your feet and practice those exercises I call the "airplane" movements. Flex your feet, circle your feet in both directions, and make figure eights going both ways with your toes and ankles engaged.

And, watching TV, what actions may make a difference? Start with having a little soft ball that you press repeatedly. If you have small weights, or even if you have two bottles of water, lift them during the commercial messages. What a workout you will have!

BONUS CHAPTER SIXTEEN HABIT: MOVE:

HAVE YOU HEARD OF NEWS REPORTS HOW ATHLETES GET THEIR BEST PHYSICAL PERFORMANCES FROM THE USE OF THEIR BRAINS? RESEARCH HAS SHOWN THAT OUR MINDS ALONE, MENTAL REHEARSAL, CAN HAVE US PERFORM AT OUR BEST.

STUDIES WITH BASKETBALL PLAYERS HAVE BEEN CONDUCTED WHERE SOME TEAM MEMBERS PRACTICE MOVES REPEATEDLY. SOME OTHER PLAYERS DO NOTHING, WHILE ANOTHER GROUP SITS AT HOME AND PRACTICES WITH THEIR MINDS ON EACH WINNING PLAY.

THE TEAM MEMBERS THAT PRACTICE ALL THE MOVES IN THEIR MIND DO THE BEST WHEN PLAYING THE ACTUAL GAME OF BASKETBALL.

SO, SIT AND VISUALIZE YOURSELF PERFORMING AT YOUR BEST AT SOME EXERCISE. CHOOSE AN EXERCISE YOU HAVE DONE BEFORE, ADD ALL FEELINGS AND SENSATIONS TO YOUR WORKOUT. ENJOY THE FEELING OF ACCOMPLISHMENT.

CHAPTER SEVENTEEN
HABIT: DECLUTTER:

Let's get really personal here. How many shirts do you own? Which shirts do you wear repeatedly? How many pairs of underwear? Which pairs fit nicely and are clean enough for that proverbial "trip to the emergency room?"

The 80/20 rule states we wear 20% of our clothing for 80% of the time. So, what are we doing with all that excess?

In 2009 I was accepted into the Unites States Peace Corps. It was a dream of mine to do this, a longer story, for another book. :-)

When faced with the reality of leaving in 2010 and renting out my home in San Diego, I choose some items to leave with dear friends, Regina and John, in Altadena. BUT, many items became excess, not anything that was essential to my happiness. And, the excess could not be added into a limited luggage allowance of the Peace Corps assignment. I realized that my memories were so much stronger than the item itself. It was fascinating to see what I stored: a few items of athletic equipment and several books of meaning. This freed me up to go and work in Ukraine. So, listen up and make decluttering you first priority.

You do not have to joint the Peace Corps to declutter! But how about you use the simplest rick of all. Place all your clothing with hangers backwards. Only if you use an item of clothing does the hanger get turned around.. At the end of a certain time, check and see which hangers have been turned, showing which items of clothing have been used.

See your time spent dressing go to a few minutes once you real-ize which items of clothing you enjoy wearing and make you feel great!

BONUS CHAPTER SEVENTEEN HABIT: DECLUTTER;

ONE OF MY FAVORITE IDEAS IS FROM THEMINIMALISTS.COM.

CHOOSE A MONTH IN WHICH TO DECLUTTER.. BEGIN ON DAY ONE AND REMOVE, DONATE, GIFT TO SOMEONE, OR THROW OUT ONE ITEM.

DAY TWO, YOU REMOVE, DONATE, GIFT, OR THROW OUT TWO ITEMS.

CONTINUE IN THIS WAY EACH DAY INCREASING THE NUMBER OF ITEMS YOU REMOVE FROM YOUR HOME. AT MONTH'S END, YOU WILL FEEL THE FREEDOM.

DO NOT REMOVE OTHER PEOPLE'S ITEMS. CONCENTRATE ON YOUR OWN BELONGINGS AS ITEMS TO BE DECLUTTERED. DO NOT BE BLINDSIDED BY "SOMEDAY I WILL NEED THIS ITEM." WE LIVE USUALLY WITHIN HALF AN HOUR DRIVE OF A STORE. WE CAN REPLACE ITEMS AT WILL.

CHAPTER EIGHTEEN HABIT: DRINK MORE WATER:

People at any age fail to drink enough water. And truly just water. Start your day with two glasses of water. Your digestion, your skin, your overall health will thank you very much.

Pleaser remove all soda and even low calorie diet soda from your drinking habits.

Also, please remove all juices from your diet.

Why? The sugar content in all soda, even the artificial sugar, cause much damage to your body. And, same with juices; they are just concentrated sugar.

Well you say, "What is left?"

You may drink coffee in moderation. You may enjoy teas, especially herbal teas and green teas. And, you may enjoy all the wonderful water you may like.

I was lucky to have a father who was an engineer for the New York City Board of Water Supply. New York City has the best rated water. You might not live close to New York City, so buy a water filter if you feel the source of your water is questionable. But, drink more water.

BONUS CHAPTER EIGHTEEN HABIT: DRINK MORE WATER;

DR. EMOTO IS A SCIENTIST WHO HAS STUDIED AND WRITTEN A NUMBER OF INTERESTING BOOKS ABOUT WATER AND HOW OUR WORDS AND THOUGHTS AFFECT THE STRUCTURE OF WATER. HIS BOOKS HAVE MANY PHOTOGRAPHS OF THE STATES OF WATER FROM HIS RESEARCH.

DR EMOTO HAS SHOWN THAT WHEN WE SEND A WORD OR THOUGHT SUCH AS LOVE OR COMPASSION TO THE DRINK OF WATER, THE MOLECULAR STRUCTURE OF THE FROZEN WATER IS MAGNIFICENTLY BEAUTIFUL IN HIS MICROSCOPIC PHOTOGRAPHS.

WHEN DR. EMOTO SENDS A WORD OR THOUGHT SUCH AS ANGER OR HATRED OR DISGUST AT THE WATER, THE STRUCTURE IN AN ELECTRON MICROSCOPE PICTURE IS DIFFERENT. DR. EMOTO DOES THIS INTENTION BY HAVING LABELS PLACED ON THE WATER. SO IF THE WORD "HATRED" OR "ANGER" IS ON THE GLASS OF WATER, THE STRUCTURE OF THE FROZEN WATER MOLECULE IS DISRUPTED AND UGLY AND MISSHAPEN.

SO, HOW ABOUT YOU LABEL YOUR WATER GLASS WITH THE WORD, "LOVE?" OR "KINDNESS' INSIDE YOUR TEA CUP WHERE YOU WILL SEE IT REPEATEDLY.

OR, IF YOUR ARE TRAINED IN REIKI, SEND REIKI ENERGY TO THE GLASS OF WATER OR THAT CUP OF TEA. ENJOY!

CHAPTER NINETEEN
HABIT: THANK YOU!:

This habit you can use any time of the day to lift your spirits and make your sense of joy shine. Be thankful for all you have! Sure, say, "But I do not have the money I want." Or, "I am feeling ill with many complaints." Or, "My job is a wreck and does not fulfill me."

We have our legs. We have our arms. We have our fingers. We have our toes. We have our heads and brains. We have our family. We have our friends. We have our homes. We have water. We have a roof over our head. Keep on going!

So, thankfulness could be just mentally done.

Or, thankfulness could be spoken out loud.

Or, thankfulness may be written down on paper or a journal of thankfulness or on typed on a computer page.

Regardless of how you express your thank yous, it is sending an energetic force of renewing your energy. And, your thank yous are increasing the energy of the whole planet. Thank you for renewing the energy!

BONUS CHAPTER NINETEEN HABIT: THANK YOU:

LET'S GO LOOK AT OUR MEMORIES. WHO WAS THE MOST INFLUENTIAL TEACHER YOU REMEMBER FROM ELEMENTARY SCHOOL?

WHO HELPED YOU THE MOST IN THE TEENAGE YEARS?

**WHO HELPED You WITH JOB OPPORTUNITIES AND JOB CHAL-
LENGES OF THE EARLY WORKING YEARS?**

**STOP AND THINK OF THE HELPFULNESS OF THOSE PEOPLE.
SEND THEM YOUR GOOD THOUGHTS RIGHT NOW. WHETHER
THESE PEOPLE ARE ALIVE OR DEAD, THE MESSSAGE WILL
REACH THEM.**

**OR, STOP RIGHT NOW AND SPEAK YOUR THANKFULNESS OUT
LOUD. TELL THIS PERSON WHAT YOU REMEMBER AND WHY
YOU ARE SO VERY THANKFUL NOW.**

**OR, WRITE A LETTER, BY HAND OR BY COMPUTER, TO SAY
THAT YOU APPRECIATE AND REMEMBER AND FEEL YOUR LIFE
CHANGED BY THEIR LOVE AND ATTENTION.**

CHAPTER TWENTY
HABIT: MEDITATE:

Ah, meditation, you have surely heard that meditation helps us in many ways with our health . Our brains are often "monkey brains." They hop from tree to tree. That is, our brains go from the past to future events again and again and leave the present moment behind..

And, you might be thinking, but meditation is just breathing, same as CHAPTER ONE HABIT. But, here's the difference: there are many different kinds of meditation. I will highlight just two kinds of meditation here. Do more research or join a group to get even more benefits.

This morning I was meditating outside on the lanai, Florida word for the porch.. I felt so good and relaxed. I felt someone there. I looked up. There was a mourning dove sitting on the roof edge and watching me directly! I laughed out loud. And the dove stayed for a long time while I felt the great benefits of sending renewing loving energy out into the energy field of the whole world .

 When we take a minute only and listen to our breathing, we allow ourselves to totally relax. If we can relax, we stop the fight or flight or freeze or foggy brain response. And we will enjoy more fun and love.

So, try this meditation, from the cat lover, me. Imagine you are sitting watching a mouse hole. Cats sit and sit so still. Imagine that as you watch that hole, thoughts start to come up. That is just a mouse coming out of the hole. Say to yourself, "That's just a thought." Then, go back to sitting and watching that mouse hole. See what else comes up. There is no need for action. There is just the sense of you begin truly aware and observant of how thoughts repeat and recycle.

Enjoy!

BONUS CHAPTER TWENTY HABIT: MEDITATE:

ONE OF MY FAVORITE ALL-TIME WEBSITES IS HEART-MATH.ORG. THEIR METHODS OF TEACHING HEART COHERENCE ARE MY FAVORITES AND HAVE HAD TREMENDOUS INFLUENCE ON MY HEALTH OVER ALL THESE YEARS.

TO REACH HEART COHERENCE, BEGIN BY PAYING ATTENTION TO YOUR BREATHING. BREATH DEEPLY AND SLOWLY.

THEN, IMAGINE THAT BREATH GOING IN AND OUT OF YOUR HEART. KEEP IMAGINING THAT ACTION. LET THE BREATH BE WHAT IS NATURAL FOR YOU.

MAKE THIS HEART-FELT FEELING EVEN STRONGER BY ALSO THINKING OF A PERSON OR PLACE THAT YOU ENJOY. MY OWN FAVORITES ARE THINKING ABOUT MY CHILDREN AND GRANDCHILDREN, OR MY DEAR SISTER TERRI.

WOW, I AM SO THANKFUL TO HAVE LEARNED ABOUT HEART-MATH.ORG IN MY 40'S. THANK YOU, THANK YOU, THANK YOU!

MORE INFORMATION:

HANKAMP.COM
SKYPE: OHANAMAGGIE

WEBSITES:
HEARTMATH.ORG
EFTUNIVERSE.COM
EMOFREE.COM
THETAPPINGSOLUTION.COM

BOOKS:

CANFIELD, JACK & PAMELA BRUNER. <u>TAPPING INTO ULTIMATE SUCCESS.</u>

CHURCH, DAWSON. <u>MIND TO MATTER.</u>

CRAIG, GARY. <u>THE EFT MANUAL.</u>

DALE, CYNDI. <u>THE SUBTLE BODY.</u>

EDEN, DONNA AND DAVID FEINSTEIN. <u>ENERGY MEDICINE.</u>

D'ERAMO, KIM. <u>THE MINDBODY TOOLBOX.</u>

GUARNERI, MIMI. <u>THE HEAT SPEAKS. 108 PEARLS.</u>

HAY, LOUISE. <u>HEAL YOUR BODY.</u>

LIPTON, BRUCE. <u>THE BIOLOGY OF BELIEF.</u>

ORTNER, NICK. <u>THE TAPPING SOLUTION.</u>

RANKIN, LISSA. <u>MIND OVER MEDICINE.</u>

RUIZ, DON MIGUEL. <u>THE FOUR AGREEMENTS.</u>

SARNOW, JOHN E. <u>HEALING BACK PAIN NATURALLY.</u>

ABOUT THE AUTHOR:

MARGARET "MAGGIE" HANKAMP is a life-long learner who reads everything, kayaks often, weeds many a garden, and enjoys working with all people.

She is a daughter and a sister and a mother and a grandmother who wishes that her children and grandchildren and whole family and friends have all the love and joy and fun that Maggie has experienced over her lifetime. Maggie continues to enjoy this love and fun and enthusiasm because she values each and every moment and each and every person.

Maggie has earned much in the way of degrees. She has a B.A. From State University at Albany, M.L.S. from Long Island University, CAS in Educational Administration from New Paltz College, and a J.D. from New York Law School.

Maggie recently earned her Massage Therapy License and is also a Reiki Teacher and Master as well as a Yoga Teacher. She especially enjoys teaching Tapping/Emotional Freedom Technique because the results are so permanent and truly amazing and FAST.

Maggie started her career learning customer service skills under Esther Ceglowski at the New York Telephone Company. Maggie became an educator and enjoyed what public libraries and later middle school students taught her about life and joy. She ran her own law firm, yet knew the world was broader and her education was just beginning. Maggie was a community development volunteer with the United States Peace Corps. She volunteered in Ukraine 2010 to 2012. She volunteered in Comoros in 2015.

Maggie returns to these countries and people "on her own dime" because of her love and respect for the friends she has met. These friends are like family and continue to teach her many things about life and joy and perseverance.

Her education continues!

Maggie wishes that you ENJOY AND LEARN AND TRY SOME NEW HABITS FOR EASY AGING!

Send her your comments at HANKAMP.@GMAI.COM.